Alkaline Ketogenic Oils For Cooking, Health & Beauty

Stimulate Healing, Lose Weight and Feel Amazing with Alkaline Keto Oils & Recipes

By Elena Garcia
Copyright Elena Garcia © 2020

All rights reserved. No part of this publication may be reproduced, stored in a retrieval system, or transmitted, in any form or by any means, electronic, mechanical, photocopying, recording or otherwise, without the prior written permission of the author and the publishers.

The scanning, uploading, and distribution of this book via the Internet or via any other means without the permission of the author are illegal and punishable by law. Please purchase only authorized electronic editions, and do not participate in or encourage electronic piracy of copyrighted materials.

Disclaimer

A physician has not written the information in this book. It is advisable that you visit a qualified dietician so that you can obtain a highly personalized treatment for your case, especially if you want to lose weight effectively. This book is for informational and educational purposes only and is not intended for medical purposes. Please consult your physician before making any drastic changes to your diet.

All information in this book has been carefully researched and checked for factual accuracy. However, the author and publishers make no warranty, expressed or implied, that the information contained herein is appropriate for every individual, situation or purpose, and assume no responsibility for errors or omission. The reader assumes the risk, and full responsibility for all actions and the author will not be held liable for any loss or damage, whether consequential, incidental, and special or otherwise, that may result from the information presented in this publication.

The book is not intended to provide medical advice or to take the place of medical advice and treatment from your personal physician. Readers are advised to consult their own doctors or other qualified health professionals regarding the treatment of medical conditions. The author shall not be held liable or responsible for any misunderstanding or misuse of the information contained in this book. The information is not intended to diagnose, treat, or cure any disease. It's merely an inspiration to live a healthy lifestyle. If you suffer from any medical condition, are pregnant, lactating, or on medication, be sure to talk to your doctor before making any drastic changes in your diet and lifestyle.

Table of Contents

Introduction 8

The Keto Super Powerful Basics 12

What Is the Alkaline Diet Craze All about? Your Body Self-Regulates Its pH So Is It Worth It? 14

    Natural & Sustainable Weight Loss 14

    All Day Energy & Healthy Glow 15

    Powerful Detox to Help You Shine & Feel Amazing 17

    The Common Mistakes with the Ketogenic Diet (Can Make You Sick and Tired While Putting the Weight Back On). 20

    The Life-Changing Role of Alkaline Foods 21

What Do Alkaline and Keto Diets Have in Common? 23

Coconut Oil Magic – The All In One Solution? 26

Coconut Oil Recipes 38

    Floral Coconut Oil Salt Scrub 39

    Sweet Dreams-Fight Insomnia Coconut Blend 40

    Easy Anti-Flu Mix 40

    Green Dream Weight Loss Smoothie 41

    Immune System Energy Smoothie 42

    Coconut Oil Cortado Style Coffee Recipe 43

    Creamy Cinnamon Latte Recipe 44

    Green Tea Weight Loss Drink 45

    Easy Creamy Warm Salmon Salad 46

    Ridiculously Easy Sweet Alkaline Keto Balls 47

Olive Oil –The Golden Oil of the Mediterranean Lifestyle 48

    Fight Cold and Flu Tea Tree Mix 51

    Sweet Dream Blend 51

    Healthy Alkaline Keto Salad Dressing 52

- Spicy Green Keto Smoothie 52
- Apple Cider Antioxidant Juice for Optimal Energy 53
- Gazpacho Celery Juice 54
- "Liver Lover" Juice 55
- Chlorophyll Spanish Gazpacho 56
- Spicy Ginger Salmon Salad 57
- On the Go Alkaline Keto Juice Shot (Liver Lover) 59

Avocado Oil – The Child of an Unusual Fruit 60
- Spicy Ginger Salmon Salad 62
- Quick Green Egg Salad 64
- Pomegranate Avocado Anti-Sugar Cravings Juice 65
- Cucumber Kale Weight Loss Juice 66
- Lime Refresher Ice Smoothie 67
- Simple Lemon Smoothie 68
- Natural Relaxation Anti-Wrinkle Blend 69
- Anti-Cellulite Blend 70

Flaxseed Oil – From Health to Skin Care 71
- Pomegranate Alkaline Green Smoothie 73
- Easy Hydration Mineral Green Smoothie 74
- Good Ol' Oil Green Smoothie 75

Brazil Nuts Quick Detox Salad 77

Easy Mediterranean Salad 78
- Easy Chilly Beetroot Soup 79

Aromatherapy & Essential Oil Recipes for Beauty & Health 80
- Water Retention Killers 80
- Beautiful Skin 81
- Acne Killers 81
- Aroma Moisturizers 82

Sesame Oil – the Ancient Ayurveda Miracle 83
Sesame Oil Recipes 86
- Tahini Sesame Energy Soup 86
- Power Sesame Smoothie 87
- Spicy Mediterranean Smoothie 88
- Mood Boosting Smoothie 89
- Healing Ashwagandha Juice 91
- Oriental Alkaline Keto Green Salad 92
- Easy Spinach'n' Nuts Salad 93
- Hair & Scalp Massage Recipe 94
- Anti-Age Sesame Oil Face Mask 94
- Ayurvedic Sesame Body Scrub 95

Introduction

Dear Reader, Thank You so much for taking an interest in this book. It means a lot to me! I wrote it to show you that living a healthy lifestyle doesn't have to be hard or complicated.

In fact, it can be as simple as learning about a few superfood oils so that you know which ones are the best for cooking, health, relaxation, or even natural beauty treatments.

Holistic health is all about *Your Inner Resourcefulness*. My number one goal is to empower you. I want to show you that it's not about some complicated health rituals or expensive supplements. True empowerment comes from a deeper understanding of the simplest (and the most effective) superfoods, such as alkaline keto oils!

Since one oil has so many different benefits, the number of healthy recipes and healthy living habits you can create is pretty much unlimited.

It's mind-blowing to discover how a few simple diet and lifestyle tweaks can radically transform your health and your life! And this book will teach you how you can make those "healthy tweaks" with alkaline ketogenic oils.

But what exactly are alkaline ketogenic (or alkaline keto) oils? Some pseudoscientific, complicated ketosis-stimulating or pH-alternating green substances? Some new online health fads? Who knows what!

Alkaline Keto Oils - Introduction

Luckily, it doesn't have to be complicated. To keep it simple, alkaline keto oils are healthy, natural oils that are good for you and for your health.
(whether you follow an alkaline diet, or a keto diet, or both, or whether you follow something else, you can always benefit from enriching your diet with some good, healthy fats!).

Some alkaline keto oils are suitable for cooking, some are an excellent choice for salads, some have the power to help you get rid of sugar and carb cravings, whereas some taste great in smoothies. Also, many of those oils can work real wonders for your skin, especially when combined with some essential oils (this book will also show you the best blends for natural, holistic beauty treatments).

So, here's precisely what you will discover in this simple, practical, no-fluff guide:

1. The basics of the alkaline and keto diets (and why it's not about changing your pH, or trying to get into some hardcore ketosis). You will also discover how you can benefit from both diets, even without being 100% perfect. In other words, you will find a few simple, yet powerful diet tweaks that will help you live a healthier lifestyle, have more energy, and, if desired, lose weight. Many people have also been able to heal their bodies and get rid of pain, inflammation, or even diabetes, just by following a more alkaline-keto friendly diet.

(While this book is not aimed at diagnosing or curing any specific health conditions, for that, you need to be talking to your doctor.

Alkaline Keto Oils - Introduction

I want to empower you and offer you the information that can at least give you some hope. Healthy eating and self-education should be your best friends on your health and wellness journey).

2. Then, I will briefly introduce you to a few powerful alkaline keto lifestyle tweaks so that you can create balance, enjoy more energy and vitality, and feel amazing!

3. You will also learn what all alkaline keto superfoods have in common and how to incorporate more of them into your diet for better health!

Finally, we will focus on the main characters of this booklet – *Alkaline Ketogenic Oils*! Each section of this book will be focusing on different oil and a variety of recipes (health, cooking, beauty, relaxation).

It's all about practical and straightforward recipes you can start experimenting with and benefiting from, even before you are done with reading this book!

So, without any further ado, let's get down to it!

Alkaline Keto Oils - Introduction

This is the 8th book in the Alkaline Keto series. The series includes:

Book 1: *Alkaline Ketogenic Mix*

Book 2: *Alkaline Ketogenic Smoothies*

Book 3: *Alkaline Ketogenic Juicing*

Book 4: *Alkaline Ketogenic Salads*

Book 5: *Alkaline Ketogenic Green Smoothies*

Book 6: *Alkaline Ketogenic Lifestyle for Massive Weight Loss*

Book 7: *Low Carb Low Sugar Smoothie Bowls*

Book 9: *Alkaline Ketogenic Superfoods*

You will find them on Amazon & our Website:

www.yourwellnessbooks.com/books

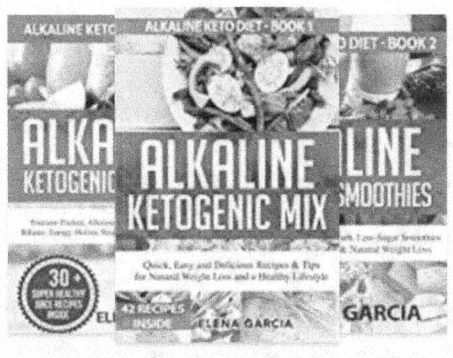

So, what exactly is the alkaline keto lifestyle? Well, it's a brilliant hybrid diet that focuses on the nourishing power of alkaline foods and the fat-burning power of keto foods. To understand how this powerful combo works, let's have a quick look at each diet.

The Keto Super Powerful Basics

To make it as simple as possible, the ketogenic diet is a diet low in carbs and high in healthy fats (and moderate in protein).

It's about reducing the carbs while adding in good, healthy fats (more on healthy vs. unhealthy fats later). This cutback in carbs puts your body into a metabolic state called ketosis.

When in ketosis, your body becomes super-efficient at burning fat for energy. A ketogenic diet can also help reduce blood sugar and insulin levels.

Transition your diet into a more keto-friendly diet. It means fewer sugars and carbs and more good fats while eating well!

Following this simple rule (even without going keto full-time) will help you transform your health and feel more energized.

The benefits of the ketogenic diet:

-it manages your sugar levels, prevents diabetes

-it normalizes your hormones and auto-immune system

-it's great for neurological health

Also, your brain will thrive. While it can use both glucose and fats for fuel, ketones are a really clean energy source. I can now concentrate much better and for much longer, while feeling less tired.

Here are other benefits of aligning your dietary choices with a ketogenic-friendly way:

-you will experience reduced hunger and reduced cravings

-you will be burning fat and reducing carbs and so normalizing your insulin levels

-you will protect your heart while raising the good cholesterol

-you will enjoy the anti-age benefits, as keto foods promote longevity and vitality (while nobody ever promised us we will live forever, by making a decision to stay healthy, we make sure that the time we are here on earth, we feel good and are vibrant).

In other words- burning crappy carbs for energy is like burning dirty fuel. However, burning fat is a much cleaner fuel while avoiding brain fog. In fact, your brain thrives on ketones.

So, here's what the ketogenic diet consists of:

-75%- 80% fat (don't worry, it's all good fat and will not make you fat).

-5-15% healthy, clean protein

-5% good, unprocessed carbs (yea, you can still eat some carbs and the carbs we will be focusing on, will be healthy unprocessed no sugar carbs so no worries, there is no starvation involved here).

The good news is that you can benefit from keto, even without doing it full-time. So many of my readers and friends have been telling me: "It all sounds great, but I don't think I could follow this diet all the time".

Well, the number one tip I can give you is – start making gradual changes. It's as simple as:

-adding more good fats into your diet (using alkaline keto oils from this book).

-reducing sugars and carbs

Rome wasn't built in a day, so don't worry about being perfect. Use the keto lifestyle philosophy as an overall health template and a slow, but a steady lifestyle change.

What Is the Alkaline Diet Craze All About? Your Body Self-Regulates Its pH So Is It Worth It?

"Going green" is the best way to describe an alkaline diet and lifestyle because the focus is on green vegetables in general, as they are the most alkaline food you can ingest.

The benefits of the alkaline diet are numerous. Let us name a few:

Natural & Sustainable Weight Loss
An alkaline diet will assist you in losing weight. One way that it does this is obvious. The foods you will be eating are very healthy, rich in minerals, and low calorie in general.

You will also be reducing the amount of acid in your body. The body stores fat to protect itself from an abundance of acid. It is a self-preservation method.

Another benefit of an alkaline lifestyle regarding weight loss is that alkaline systems have more oxygen in their cells. Oxygen is an essential part of eliminating fat cells from the body. The more oxygen in your system, the more efficient your metabolism will be.

All Day Energy & Healthy Glow

Going green does not only give you energy for the apparent reason that you are eating many more healthy, energizing vitamins. You are negating the acid-induced lethargy that is brought on by an unhealthy acid-forming diet.

Not only do our bodies need an abundance of oxygen to lose weight, but we also need oxygen in our cells to energize us. The lack of oxygen in our cells causes fatigue. No, it is not just because you worked too late or partied too hard the night before. It is internal. If your cells are trying to function in a highly acidic environment, they will not be able to transfer oxygen efficiently; leading of course to exhaustion.

Cells in the body also make something that is called adenosine triphosphate (ATP). If your system is very acidic, it harms the ability of your cells to produce it. In the scientific world, it is known as the "energy currency of life." The ATP molecule contains the energy that we need to accomplish most things that we do (both internally and externally).

BODILY FUNCTIONS

Another benefit of the alkaline lifestyle is that your body will be able to function at an optimum level instead of being inhibited by acids:

- Your heartbeat is thrown off by acidic wastes in the body. The stomach suffers greatly from over-acidity.

- The liver's job is to get rid of acid toxins, but also to produce alkaline enzymes. By simply reducing your acid intake, you can internally boost your alkalinity thanks to your liver!

- Your pancreas thrives on alkalinity. Too much acid in your system throws off your pancreas. If you eat alkaline foods, your pancreas can regulate your blood sugars.

- Your kidneys also help to keep your body alkaline. When they are overwhelmed by an acidic diet, they cannot do their job.

- The lymph fluids function most efficiently in an alkaline system. They remove acid waste. Acidic systems not only have a slower lymph flow causing acids to be stored; they can also cause acids to be reabsorbed through lymphatic ducts in your intestines that would typically be excreted.

Powerful Detox to Help You Shine & Feel Amazing

Another huge benefit of an alkaline lifestyle is detoxification. First, you are going to be cutting out processed foods that are continually adding toxins to your system.

Secondly, you are going to be eating foods that allow your body to detox and rid itself of the acids that have built up in your system all this time. When we detoxify our bodies, our emotions, bodily functions, and mental functions are able to operate at their optimal levels.

The number of benefits that come with living alkaline are numerous. As you help your body rebalance its optimal blood pH, you will find, as I did, that you have never felt better. I am still seeing improvement and reaping the rewards of this holistic approach to not only eating alkaline foods but living alkaline.

Our bodies function optimally when our blood is at about 7.365 - 7.45 pH.

The alkaline <u>diet is not about changing or "raising" your pH</u>. This is where many alkaline guides go wrong. You see, our body is smart enough to **self-regulate** our pH for us, no matter what we eat.

Unfortunately, when you constantly bombard your body with acid-forming foods (for example, processed foods, fast food, alcohol, sugar, and even too much meat) you torture your body with incredible stress. Why? Well, because it has to work harder to maintain that optimal pH...

Here's a very simple example...

Imagine you immerse yourself in a bath filled with ice. You say, but hey, my body can self-regulate its optimal temperature, right? And yes, it can. But it will eventually collapse, and you will get ill. The same happens with nutrition and our blood pH.

You can spend years indulging in toxic, processed, acid-forming foods that only deprive your body of its vital nutrients, saying: "But hey, my body will self-regulate its optimal blood pH."

And again, it will...but sooner or later it will give up and manifest a disease. It will accumulate fat as its natural defense function to protect your body from over-acidity. We don't wanna end up there, right?

So, to sum up- the alkaline diet is a natural, holistic system, a nutritional lifestyle that advocates the consumption of fresh, unprocessed foods that are rich in alkaline nutrients. These are called alkaline foods, and they help your body stimulate its optimal healing functions. Yes! A healthy body needs nutrients, and fresh low sugar fruits and vegetables are great for that.

Shifting your diet to one that is full of alkaline foods is one of the easiest and best things you can do for your overall health. And the best thing is- we will be combining alkaline foods with keto-friendly meals to make it easy, delicious and fun! Much simpler to follow for the long term.

But the way we see it is this- it's perfect! Plus, it's not a diet; it's a lifestyle.

What I like about the alkaline diet is that you don't have to be 100% perfect. It's enough to make sure you add a ton of greens and veggies and make your diet rich in alkaline foods.

It's easy to do when you focus on serving your lunch or dinner with a big green salad or start drinking green juices with alkaline keto oils (the recipe section will show you how).

Alkaline Keto Basics – the Holistic Approach to Health

When it comes to the alkaline diet, there is something called the 70/30 rule meaning that about 70% of your diet should be fresh, nutrient-dense alkaline-forming foods and the remaining 30% can be acid- forming foods (however they still should be clean and organic, for example, grass-fed meat or organic eggs).This is what a hybrid alkaline keto lifestyle is all about. Healthy greens, vegetables, quality animal products, and good fats.

Simple. Balanced. Flexible. Common-sense!

While this book focuses on oils, we have created a printable alkaline keto food lists to help you on your journey. To get our recommended alkaline keto food lists, visit our private website at:

www.yourwellnessbooks.com/alkalineketo

The alkaline keto food lists will help you identify which foods you should be eating more off so that you can feel confident knowing you are getting closer to your wellness and weight loss goals.

(any problems with your download, please email: info@yourwellnessbooks.com)

The Common Mistakes with the Ketogenic Diet (Can Make You Sick and Tired While Putting the Weight Back On).

The most common mistake that people make is that they do not include enough veggies with their keto foods. That can cause imbalance and acidity. Hence, I am such a big fan of keto and alkaline diets combined. Green vegetables are a fantastic addition to your keto diet.

They will help you have more energy and also add more variety to your diet.

The real keto lifestyle is about variety, abundance, and energy. It's hard to be successful with a keto diet if a menu consists entirely of animal products.

The Life-Changing Role of Alkaline Foods

It's important to get a ton of greens, and alkaline foods as these foods are rich in minerals and vitamins while at the same time don't contain sugar.

I have been promoting alkaline foods for years.

They oxygenate your body and help you have more energy and can be combined with other diets such as paleo or keto diet.

In its optimal design, alkaline diet advocates using quality plant-based oils such as avocado and olive oil, and coconut oil, and it also excludes wheat products and crappy carbs.

Foods that are rich in sugar are also excluded. The alkaline diet includes low sugar fruits (limes, lemons, grapefruits etc.)

One of the main principles of the alkaline diet is adding a ton of green veggies into your diet.

The best way to be adding these alkaline foods is via veggie smoothies and juices. The recipe section of this book will give you some ideas. There are also many fantastic alkaline-friendly drinks that will not only help you re-energize and alkalize your body without messing around with your keto lifestyle but will also bring more variety into your diet. Many of these drinks will help you feel more relaxed and balanced.

They will also help you quit drinking sugary drinks, and soda's and, in many cases, can also help you reduce your caffeine intake. It's a great feeling if you can just wake up and go without depending on caffeine and sugar and feeling moody all the time.

Alkaline Keto Basics – the Holistic Approach to Health

Be sure to get your printable alkaline keto food lists for extra study:

www.yourwellnessbooks.com/alkalineketo

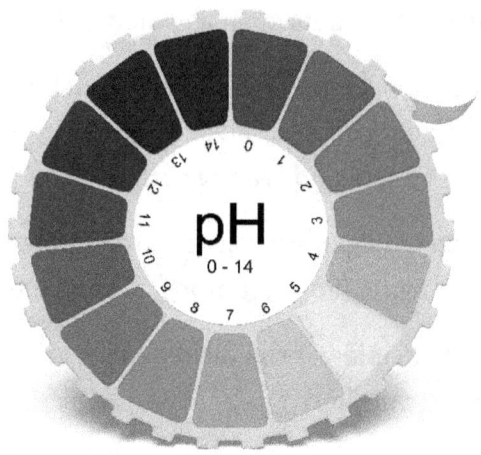

What Do Alkaline and Keto Diets Have in Common?

Even though at first sight, alkaline and keto diets may seem to be very different, there are also many similarities. For example:

-both diets stay away from all forms of sugar, even fructose (hence both alkaline and keto diets focus on low sugar fruit).

-both diets stay away from processed carbs, gluten, and wheat

-both diets like leafy greens and veggies

-both diets like good fats and healthy oils

Which brings us to the meat and potatoes of this book. Alkaline keto oils! First of all, let's have a look at which oils to avoid. This little tweak alone can really benefit your and your family's health.

Oils to avoid:

-industrial seed oil, trans-fatty acid

- industrial vegetable oils- they are very processed, very corrosive to our arteries, they produce heart disease

-Soybean oil

-Sunflower oil

-Cottonseed oil

-Corn oil

-Canola oil (rapeseed oil)

Condiments like mayonnaise also contain the above-mentioned toxic oils, and so do industrially made bakes and goods.

The fast-food industry uses those oils too.

Instead, you want to focus on healthy, alkaline ketogenic oils, such as:

-coconut oil

-olive oil

-avocado oil

-flaxseed oil

-sesame oil

Personally, my favorite oils are coconut oil (for cooking and healthy keto fat bombs or no-cook desserts), olive oil (for salads, for veggie smoothies, or certain types of traditional Mediterranean cuisine), and avocado oil (also for salads and all kinds of smoothies).

These are my personal choices. However, I also enjoy learning about and experimenting with other oils, such as sesame oil and flaxseed oil. When it comes to purchasing those oils, you don't need to have all of them. Just get started on one or two (for example, one for cooking and one for salads).

While I don't want to come across as biased, coconut oil is probably the universal oil, one that works very well for cooking as well as many other recipes (beauty, relaxation, smoothies, weight loss, healing and more). The only downside is, it's not really possible to use it in salads (here's where olive oil comes in very handy).

All the oils recommended in this book can be purchased quite inexpensively on Amazon.

We have listed a few recommended brands and deals on our private website, in case you want to check it out and save your time:

www.YourWellnessBooks.com/oils

So, without further ado, let's learn more about each alkaline keto oil, what it's suitable for as well as a myriad of super healthy recipes for health, cooking, healing, and beauty!

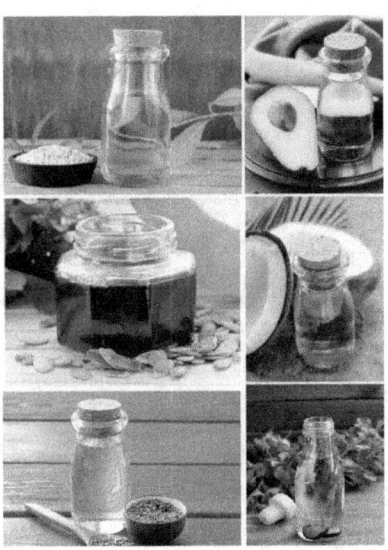

Coconut Oil Magic – The All In One Solution?

Coconut oil is probably the most famous oil out there. It has been called a superfood and miracle oil many times. And, as a Celebrity Oil, it surely lives up to its expectations!

Its unique combination of fatty acids has many health benefits such as boosting fat loss, improving heart health, and brain function.

Coconut oil has numerous wellness powers, such as:

1. Healthy fatty acids

Coconut oil is very rich in certain saturated fats that have very positive effects on the body:

-They can stimulate fat burn while providing a quick energy boost. -They raise HDL (good) cholesterol in your blood (some studies say that HDL may help reduce heart disease risk.)

So, what is the difference between most dietary fats and coconut oil?

Most dietary fats are categorized as long-chain triglycerides (LCTs). Coconut oil, on the other hand, contains some medium-chain triglycerides (MCTs), which are shorter fatty acid chains.

When you eat medium-chain triglycerides (MCTs), they go straight to your liver. Then, your body can automatically use them as a quick source of energy (it can also turn them into ketones).

Ketones are especially beneficial for your brain. Many studies point to ketones as a possible treatment for epilepsy, Alzheimer's disease, and other medical conditions.

2. Improved heart health

Coconut oil is one of the most popular health foods in the Western World. But, it's still relatively new in our culture, and we surely haven't been consuming it for hundreds of years. The question is – what could be the long-term benefits of using coconut oil regularly?

Well, a fascinating fact is that some countries have been using coconut oil as one of the main "staple foods" in their diets. Many people living in those countries have been using coconut oil for generations. An example of that are the people of a small island chain in the South Pacific, called Tokelau. Most of them obtained about 60% of their calories from coconuts and coconut oil. The heart disease rate in Tokealu was extremely low, and most people enjoyed a good overall health.

Was it because of the coconut only? Could other factors and lifestyle choices influence that as well? Perhaps, it's their genetics?

Well, it's up to you to make your decision. For me, it's one of the examples of how coconut oil can positively influence our health if we choose to use it.

Another example, similar to the Tokelau islands, are Kitavan people in Papua, New Guinea. They also eat a lot of coconuts (as well as fresh fruit and fish) and hardly ever suffer from heart disease. Once again, this could also be due to the climate, genetics, and other foods they consume as well as their overall healthy, natural, and real food lifestyle. However, the one thing they have in common is that they have been consuming coconut and coconut oil for generations.

3. A fat that burns fat?

I talk to my readers and newsletter subscribers regularly. They all have different health goals they wish to reach. However, the number one health goal that most of the people I talk to wish to accomplish is weight loss and fat burn. And even those who have already reached their weight loss goals, still continue their "healthy weight loss" journey because they want to maintain the results of their effort and hard work.

The interesting thing is that some people think weight loss or weight gain is just a matter of how many calories we eat. While there is some truth to that calories in and out theory (and it makes sense), the source of the calories is very important too. You see, different foods affect your body and your hormones in different ways. For example, you could eat 2000 processed calories from an unhealthy fast-food meal that satisfies your dopamine levels for a short period of time (while leaving your body malnourished and hungry, not to mention the damage caused by all the chemicals, processed sugars, and carbs from fast food). Or, you could eat 2000 calories from a healthy, clean food source to feed and nourish your body and create balance so that you no longer crave processed sugars, and weight loss becomes easier.

You see, the already mentioned, miraculous MCTs in coconut oil can speed up the number of calories your body burns compared with longer-chain fatty acids.

Aside from that, coconut oil is a clean, healthy, and natural food. As such, it offers clean, healthy, natural, and unprocessed calories.

Word of caution, though. Some people treat coconut oil as a health and weight loss shortcut. What I mean by that is an exaggeration. You hear some food is good for you and so you overdo it to get the results fast. Well, common-sense should be your best friend! Coconut oil, by itself, will not work wonders on your health and life. It's all about changing your lifestyle, eating a clean food diet, and moving your body. Then, use coconut oil as a natural supplement, for example, have a tablespoon of coconut oil when craving sugar or processed sweets. Or add some to your smoothies (more in the recipe section).

Also remember, even the healthiest superfood can harm you if you overdo it or try to use it as a shortcut. And yes, it is high in calories.

So, for some people, it can lead to weight gain if eaten in large amounts (and from a place of "I don't want to change my diet and lifestyle, I just want some new superfood to work wonders for me").

We will come back to weight loss with coconut oil later in the recipe section. However, if weight loss is your goal, I highly recommend you read my book: *Alkaline Ketogenic Lifestyle for Massive Weight Loss* (Alkaline Keto Diet book #6) which you can order from Amazon (Kindle and paperback, audio coming soon). It's a short read, but it's very to the point. It will help you determine what to focus on to lose weight and keep it off, without sacrificing your health, hormone balance, and sanity.

Now, let's get back to the wellness powers of coconut oil.

4. Antimicrobial effects of coconut oil thanks to lauric acid?

About 50% of the fatty acids in coconut oil are made of lauric acid.

You see, when your body digests lauric acid, it creates a unique substance called monolaurin.

Now, both lauric acid and monolaurin have been proven to have the ability to kill harmful pathogens, such as bacteria, viruses, and fungi. Thanks to this fantastic benefit, many people (including myself) have turned to coconut oil as a mouthwash.

While there is no clear scientific evidence that coconut oil reduces your risk of flu, internal infections or the common cold, personally, I feel very empowered knowing the benefits of the lauric acid and have been getting fewer infections after I started using coconut oil (both as a mouthwash and internally).

I always say – if something works for you, keep on doing it! Also, coconut oil is still relatively new in our society. While many people have reported numerous health benefits after using coconut oil, science needs much more data and time to turn people's health successes into a reliable scientific report (this is my personal take on it).

So, to sum up, while using coconut oil as a mouthwash may prevent mouth infections and many people have been using it successfully as a natural, chemical-free healthy ritual, more evidence is needed to back it up.

5.Reduced hunger and sugar/carb cravings.

"Elena, whenever you crave sugar or carbs, or anything unhealthy, just have a tablespoon of the coconut oil, it will do the trick for you" – this is what my alkaline nutrition teacher told me way before I learned about the benefits of coconut oil.

Back then, I thought it was crazy! But boy, did it work!

Now, this is exactly what I recommend to my readers and subscribers.

So, how does it work with coconut oil as a hunger suppressant?

One exciting feature of MCTs is that they may reduce hunger.

This may be related to the way your body metabolizes fats, because ketones can reduce a person's appetite. Many people have reported that eating 1-2 tablespoons of coconut oil in the morning, not only helps them avoid mid-morning hunger and sugar cravings, but it also helps make healthier lunch choices. My personal theory behind it is that health attracts health. One healthy choice can lead to another.

6. Healthy skin, hair, and teeth

Coconut oil can also be used for cosmetic purposes and natural beauty treatments. It has been scientifically proven that coconut oil improves the moisture content of dry skin. It can also reduce the symptoms of eczema.

Coconut oil is also great for holistic hair treatments. Massage your hair and scalp with coconut oil and keep the oil in for at least one hour. Then, wash your hair with a gentle shampoo.

Many people use coconut oil as a natural sunscreen. However, it's not entirely safe, as the studies confirmed it could only block about 20% of the sun's ultraviolet (UV) rays.

Another exciting natural beauty therapy with coconut oil is the already mentioned oil pulling.

Oil pulling involves swishing coconut oil in your mouth like mouthwash to improve dental hygiene while reducing bad breath.

7. Less harmful abdominal fat.

As we already learned, some of the fatty acids in coconut oil can reduce appetite and increase fat burning, while leading to healthy and natural weight loss.

Abdominal fat (also called: visceral fat) loves "hanging out" in the abdominal cavity as well as around your organs. MCTs from coconut oil have shown to be especially effective at reducing belly fat.

The simple lifestyle change you can make is to replace your other cooking fats with healthy coconut oil, which brings us to the next benefit of coconut oil.

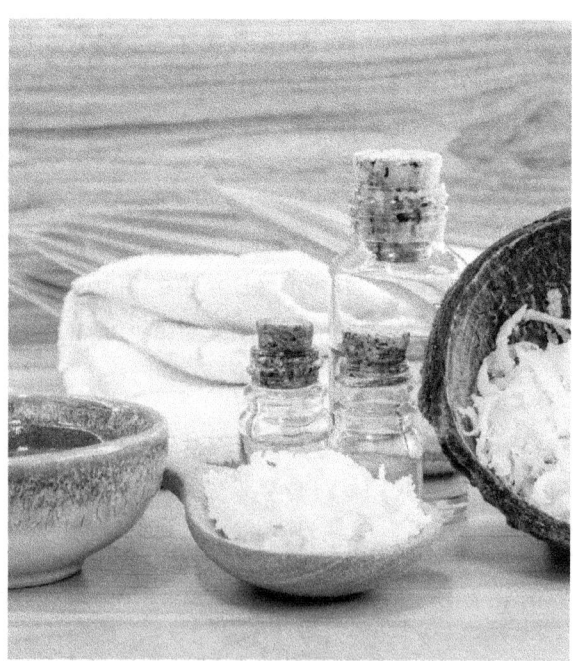

8. Safe cooking even at high temperatures.

About 87% of coconut oil is saturated fat. This amazing feature makes it one of the healthiest oils for high-heat cooking, as well as frying.

What makes saturated fats so unique is that unlike the polyunsaturated fatty acids found in vegetable oils (such as sunflower, canola oil, corn, or safflower) they retain their structure even when heated to high temperatures.

The reason why some vegetable oils are so unhealthy is that they are converted into toxic compounds when heated.

Luckilly, coconut oil is a fully holistic and natural oil for cooking even at high temperatures. It also makes your food taste great and smells fantastic!

9. Skin Irritation Relief & Natural Eczema Treatment

Coconut oil has been proven to offer a natural healing solution for dermatitis and other skin disorders. Another benefit is that while most commercially produced creams and moisturizes are very expensive, coconut oil can be a simple and affordable solution.

10. Better Focus and Brain Function

Coconut oil can be a great alternative energy source for your brain as the MCT in coconut oil and easily broken down by your liver and then turned into ketons.

11. Natural Stain Remover

Surprisingly enough, coconut oil can be also used to get rid of stains, as well as spills on carpets and furniture.

Simply combine coconut oil with baking soda (1:1 proportion) and then mix into a paste. Apply the paste the stain and wipe away after 8 minutes.

12. Natural Deodorant

Coconut oil is full of strong antibacterial properties, therefore, making it an excellent natural deodorant with no nasty chemicals.

A simple recipe is to add one drop of tea tree essential oil to one teaspoon of coconut oil and apply it as a deodorant.

13. Quick & Natural Energy Source

If drinking too much coffee makes you feel anxious, try some coconut oil. As you already know, coconut oil contains medium-chain triglyceride fatty acids, and these are digested very differently than the long-chain triglycerides found in most foods.

The medium-chain triglyceride fatty acids go directly from your gut to your liver, to be used as a quick source of energy that won't make you nervous like caffeine does (and it won't raise blood sugar levels like sugar or carbs).

14. Natural Eye Makeup Remover

Coconut oil is a natural and inexpensive way to remove your make-up. It's also very gentle to the eyes. Apply it with a cotton pad, like a regular make-up remover, and wipe gently until your make-up is removed.

15. Natural Lip Balm

Coconut oil is perfect as a natural lip moisturizer. Not only will it leave your lips moist for hours, but it will also provide some sun protection too.

16. Hormone support

Getting the wrong kinds of fats can create havoc on hormones. Coconut oil contains specific fats that support the body's natural hormone production.

So now, let's have a look at different kinds of coconut oil so that you know which one to buy.

Unrefined Organic Coconut Oil

This type of oil offers the best of the benefits listed above. It is extracted from fresh coconut. Since only a wet-milled fermentation process is used, the beneficial properties of the coconut remain untouched. This exact type of coconut oil has been proven to have the highest antioxidant levels. Even though this process does use heat, the studies show that it does not harm the oil or reduce nutrient levels.

"Extra Virgin" Coconut Oil

"Extra Virgin" is an excellent standard for olive oil but not for coconut oil. This is produced by cold-pressing the oil, and this process does not preserve the antioxidants as well.

Refined Coconut Oils

Refined coconut oil is usually tasteless and has no coconut smell. It is very often heated, bleached, and deodorized. Even though healthy options are available, many refined coconut oils do not have the benefits of unrefined.

Fractionated Oil or MCT Oil

Fractionated oil or MCT oil is liquid coconut oil. What makes it different from unrefined oils is that it does not get solid below 76 degrees. Unfortunately, it doesn't contain all of the beneficial properties of unrefined coconut oil.

What Type of Coconut Oil to Use?

For external uses (hair or skincare) expeller-pressed, fractionated, or other types of refined coconut oil are fine, but for internal use, unrefined organic oil is best.

You will find our personal recommendations and oil brands at:

www.YourWellnessBooks.com/oils

Now, let's have a look at some amazing coconut oil recipes!

Olive Oil Secrets

Coconut Oil Recipes

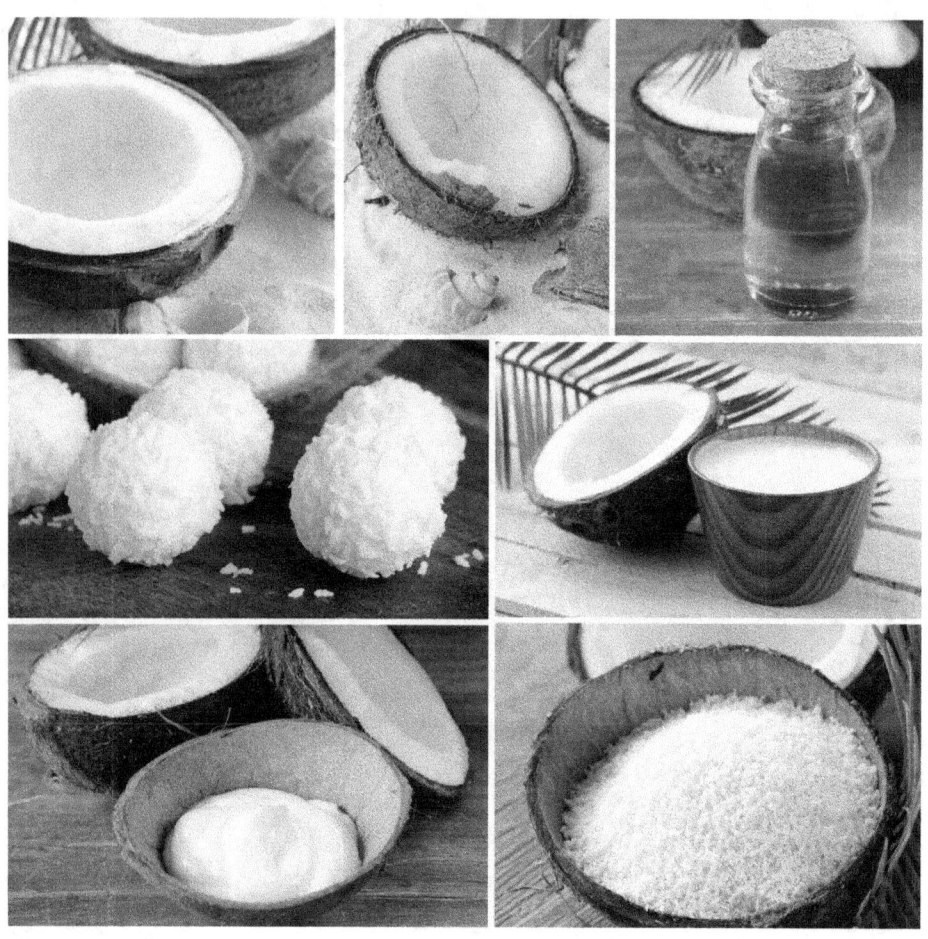

Floral Coconut Oil Salt Scrub

This floral coconut oil salt scrub is made with just a few simple ingredients, but it will leave your skin feeling fresh and clean. Use it daily for the best results!

Ingredients:

- 2 cups cold-pressed coconut oil
- 1 cup Epsom salt
- 10 drops jasmine essential oil
- 10 drops lavender essential oil

Instructions:

1. Combine the coconut oil, Epsom salt, and essential oils in a mixing bowl.
2. Stir the ingredients until thoroughly combined.
3. Spoon the mixture into a glass jar and cover tightly with the lid.
4. When ready to use, dampen your skin then apply a small amount of the scrub.
5. Gently rub the scrub into your skin in a circular motion, then rinse and pat dry.

Sweet Dreams-Fight Insomnia Coconut Blend

Blend:

- 2 tablespoons of coconut oil
- 2 drops of lavender essential oil
- 2 drops of fennel essential oil

Add to your bath or use for self-massage.

Easy Anti-Flu Mix

Blend:

- 2 tablespoons of coconut oil
- 2 drops of eucalyptus essential oil
- 2 drops of tea tree essential oil

Add to your Epsom salt bath or use for self-massage.

Green Dream Weight Loss Smoothie

This green vegetable smoothie blends the best of the alkaline and keto worlds. It's my number one recommendation if your goal is weight loss. It may take some time to get used to green vegetable smoothies. Especially, if you are more accustomed to drinking "sweety-carby-fruity" smoothies (not that good for you, unfortunately).

But trust me, after a few green smoothies, and fantastic energy they provide, you will be wondering how you could ever live without them.

Servings: 2

Ingredients:

- 1 cup coconut or almond milk (unsweetened)
- 1 cup water (filtered, preferably alkaline)
- 1 small avocado, peeled and pitted
- A handful of spinach
- 2 tablespoons coconut oil
- Pinch of Himalaya salt to taste

Instructions:

1. Place all the ingredients in a blender.
2. Blend well.
3. Serve and enjoy!

Immune System Energy Smoothie

This is a super simple alkaline green smoothie that will help you boost your immune system by enriching your diet with vitamin C and a myriad of alkaline minerals.

Serves 1-2

Ingredients

- 2 big limes, peeled
- 1 cup of coconut or almond milk
- A handful of kale leaves, washed
- Optional- a few drops of liquid chlorophyll
- 1 lime wedge to garnish (1 per serving)
- 1-2 tablespoons coconut oil
- 1 teaspoon cinnamon powder
- Stevia to sweeten, if needed

Instructions

1. Place in a blender.
2. Process until smooth.
3. Serve in a smoothie glass and garnish with a wedge of lime.
4. Enjoy!

Coconut Oil Cortado Style Coffee Recipe

This recipe is perfect if you are not a breakfast person!

Ingredients:
- 1 expresso
- 1 tablespoon coconut oil
- 2-4 tablespoons coconut milk

Instructions:
1. Combine all the ingredients in a small coffee cup.
2. Mix well, drink, and enjoy!

Creamy Cinnamon Latte Recipe

Cinnamon makes this coffee taste so nice, and it also prevents sugar cravings- we always want to tackle the problem from different angles!

Ingredients:
- 1 cup coconut milk, warm
- 1 expresso
- 2 tablespoons coconut oil
- 1 teaspoon cinnamon

Stevia to sweeten, if needed (it's a natural ingredient, it's not processed, and it has no sugar in it- the perfect addition to your drinks and smoothies if you like it sweet).

Instructions:
1. Blend all the ingredients in a hand blender.
2. Shake well, serve, and enjoy!

Green Tea Weight Loss Drink

This simple tea-based drink is perfect as a quick afternoon pick me up!

Ingredients:
- 1 cup of green tea
- 1 cup coconut milk
- 2 tablespoons coconut oil
- Stevia to sweeten if needed

Instructions:
Blend all the ingredients, serve, and enjoy!

Easy Creamy Warm Salmon Salad

Salmon is one of my favorite keto ingredients, especially to use for quick, nourishing salads like this one.

Servings: 1-2

Ingredients:

- Half cup raw cashews, crushed
- 4 slices of smoked salmon
- 2 tablespoons of coconut oil
- 1 cup fresh spinach
- 2 tomatoes, sliced
- Himalaya salt and black pepper to taste
- A few thin slices of cheddar cheese

Instructions:

1. Place coconut oil in a frying pan.
2. Switch on the heat (medium heat).
3. Add the spinach and Himalaya salt and stir-fry until soft.
4. Now, add the salmon, cashews, and tomato slices.
5. Stir fry until the salmon is warm.
6. Take off the heat and place in a salad bowl.
7. If needed, add more Himalaya salt to taste.
8. Top up with some cheddar cheese, serve and enjoy!

Olive Oil Secrets

Ridiculously Easy Sweet Alkaline Keto Balls

This recipe is a must-try to help you:

-satisfy your "sweet tooth" without eating crappy carbs or sugars

-add in some good fats and anti-inflammatory properties too

-sneak in some alkaline keto superfoods to make sure you stay energized

Ingredients:

- 1 cup raw cashews (unsalted, unsweetened), soaked for at least 4 hours
- 1 cup raw almonds (unsalted, unsweetened), soaked for at least 4 hours
- 4 tablespoons coconut oil
- 4 tablespoons coconut milk
- 1 tablespoon cinnamon powder

Instructions:

1. Place all the ingredients in a high-speed blender or a food processor.
2. Using your hands, form the "dough" into small balls.
3. Place the balls on a big plate and put them in a fridge for a few hours.
4. Serve and enjoy!

Now, let's have a look at olive oil….

Olive Oil – The Golden Oil of the Mediterranean Lifestyle

Olive oil is an integral component of the Mediterranean diet. It is very abundant in healing antioxidants. The main fat it contains is a monounsaturated fatty acids (considered to be a healthy fat).

The antioxidants in olive oil offer protection from cellular damage, therefore, minimizing the risk of different health conditions and diseases. Extra virgin olive oil has a more bitter flavor, however, it contains more antioxidants than other kinds of olive oil, as it undergoes the least processing.

Olive oil is made from olives, the fruit of the olive tree, and a traditional crop of the Mediterranean region.

You can use olive oil for cooking, cosmetics, medicine, and even soaps. Traditionally it is also used for pizza and pasta as well as a salad dressing.

The main benefits of olive oil:

-extra virgin olive oil helps prevent cellular damage caused by free radicals (because of its high antioxidant content)

-it's very good for a healthy cardiovascular system

People who eat a Mediterranean diet, and consume olive oil daily, seem to have a higher life expectancy, compared to people who eat processed food and fast food diet. Many Mediterranean experts call it "the standard in preventive medicine."

- olive oil used might reduce inflammation, blood sugar, and triglycerides (fats in the blood), as well as the "bad" cholesterol. At the same time, it can increase levels of high-density lipoprotein (HDL), also called the "good" cholesterol.

- some scientists even suggest that including extra virgin olive oil in your diet may help prevent Alzheimer's disease (because of its protective impact on blood vessels in the brain).

- molecules in extra virgin olive oil may help prevent or repair liver damage. In fact, many Mediterranean naturopathic recipes recommend juice of one lemon mixed with 1 tablespoon of olive oil as a natural remedy to strengthen the liver.

- phenols found in olive oil may also help boost intestinal immunity and gut health by changing the microbes in the gut, therefore helping people who have colitis and other types of IBD.

- Olive oil is very rich in fat-soluble vitamins A, D, E, and K, making it a highly precious, natural skin moisturizer. For better results, you can mix 1 tablespoon of olive oil with 2 drops of lavender essential oil. Use as a face and neck moisturizer before going to bed.

- Olive oil is a proven, natural after-sun treatment. It will make your skin smooth and hydrated.

- You can also use it as a natural body scrub by mixing it with some Epsom salt and a few drops of a chosen essential oil.

- Just like coconut oil, olive oil can also be used as a natural makeup remover. You can also use it as a natural face mask (some secret beauty hacks from my Mediterranean grandma – olive oil mixed with egg whites and honey can work real wonders for your skin! It is also an excellent, all-natural wrinkle treatment).

However, be sure you only use quality, organic oils, and first test a small portion of your skin to see if you don't have an allergic reaction.

How to buy the best olive oil?

Be sure to choose an extra virgin olive oil, as it's much less processed and therefore retains its powerful antioxidant content.

Also, it's good to note that extra virgin olive oil has a high smoke point of 376 °F (191°C), so it is safe to use for most cooking methods. However, when people fry in olive oil for a long time, this can lead to degradation of the fats and the production of toxic compounds. So, if cooking with olive oil, use it for quick sautéing or frying and do not use it for prolonged frying methods, to keep it healthy.

Now, let's have a look at some olive oil recipes!

Fight Cold and Flu Tea Tree Mix

You need:

-1 tablespoon of olive oil

-2 drops of tea tree essential oil (suitable for internal use, be sure to double-check because not all essential oil brands are safe to ingest; the brand I always use is Pranarom).

Combine the olive oil with tea tree oil. Take before going to bed, to strengthen your immune system, or whenever you feel like you are catching a cold. You can also use it for prevention (but for any extended uses, be sure to talk to a naturopathic doctor).

Sweet Dream Blend

Combine 1 tablespoon of olive oil with 2 drops of lavender essential oil (suitable for internal use, I use Pranarom lavender essential oil). Have this mix before you go to bed or whenever you need to relax.

Healthy Alkaline Keto Salad Dressing

This simple salad dressing is all-natural and full of healing nutrients. It can really make your salads taste amazing!

Ingredients:

-juice of 1 lime or lemon

-Half teaspoon Himalaya salt

-half teaspoon Italian spices

-4 tablespoons olive oil

Blend and use for your favorite healthy salads!

Spicy Green Keto Smoothie

This simple smoothie is a super simple energy booster, and it also helps prevent sugar cravings.

Ingredients:

-1 big avocado, peeled and pitted

-1 small chili flake

-pinch of Himalayan salt

-Juice of 1 lime

-2 tablespoons olive oil

-half cup water, filtered

Instructions:

Blend and enjoy!

Apple Cider Antioxidant Juice for Optimal Energy

This recipe is full of miraculous nutrients to help you get rid of toxins. Its therapeutic properties are enhanced by Apple Cider Vinegar.

Servings: 1-2
Ingredients:
- 2 cucumbers, peeled and sliced
- Half cup of celery leaves
- Half cup of mint leaves
- 2 tablespoons of olive oil
- 1 tablespoon apple cider vinegar (organic)
- Himalayan salt to taste (optional)

Instructions:
1. Juice all the ingredients.
2. Add in the olive oil, apple cider vinegar, Himalayan salt, and black pepper (optional)
3. Serve and enjoy!

Gazpacho Celery Juice

This recipe tastes a bit like Spanish gazpacho and can get you hooked on celery.

Serves: 1
Ingredients:
- 2 big tomatoes
- 2 big cucumbers, peeled
- 4 celery sticks, chopped
- 1 tablespoon olive oil
- Himalayan salt and black pepper to taste

Instructions:
1. Juice all the ingredients.
2. Add in olive oil, Himalayan salt, and black pepper.
3. Stir well, serve and enjoy!

"Liver Lover" Juice

Grapefruits are very rich in phytonutrients called limonoids that promote the production of antioxidant enzymes. These help the liver to remove toxic compounds easier, thereby protecting the liver in the process.

Servings: 2
Ingredients:
- 2 grapefruits, peeled
- 1 inch of fresh root ginger, peeled
- Half cup water, filtered, preferably alkaline
- Pinch of Himalayan salt
- 2 tablespoons of olive oil

Instructions:
1. Juice all the ingredients.
2. Add the water, Udo's Choice, Himalayan salt, and olive or avocado oil.
3. Stir well and drink to your health.

Chlorophyll Spanish Gazpacho

This recipe is a variation of the original Spanish gazpacho recipe in a super alkaline keto green version.

Serves: 2

Ingredients

- 3 medium-sized cucumbers, peeled and chopped
- 1 green bell pepper
- 1 big garlic clove, peeled
- 2 tablespoons extra-virgin, cold-pressed olive oil
- 1 cup filtered water
- Half cup almond milk
- Pinch of Himalayan salt
- Pinch of black pepper

Instructions

1. Place all the ingredients in a blender and process until smooth.
2. Serve in a smoothie glass and enjoy!
3. If you prefer to enjoy this recipe as a soup, you can garnish it with some chopped veggies, herbs, and spices.
4. Enjoy!

Spicy Ginger Salmon Salad

Ginger is well-known for its anti-inflammatory and healing properties. Cucumbers are highly refreshing and very alkaline-forming. Salmon, avocado, nuts, and healthy oils will help you stay full for hours!

Serves: 2
Ingredients
For the Salad:
- 2 cucumbers, peeled and thinly sliced
- 1 tablespoon of grated ginger
- 1 cup arugula leaves
- 1 big avocado, peeled, pitted and sliced
- A handful of crushed almonds
- 2 slices of smoked salmon, cut into smaller pieces

For the Dressing:
- 1 tablespoon olive oil
- 1 tablespoon avocado oil
- 1 tablespoon fresh lime juice
- Black pepper to taste
- Himalayan salt to taste

To garnish:
- A few orange wedges
- A handful of cilantro leaves

Instructions:
1. Combine all the salad ingredients in a big salad bowl and toss well.
2. Mix all the salad dressing ingredients. You can use a small hand blender, or quickly combine and stir all the ingredients in a small bowl.
3. Pour the dressing over the salad and toss well.
4. Sprinkle over a handful of cilantro leaves and garnish with orange wedges.
5. Serve and enjoy!

On the Go Alkaline Keto Juice Shot (Liver Lover)

This recipe is perfect if you are too busy to juice...
You know...setting up the juicer, cleaning up.
Well, this recipe doesn't even need a proper juicer. A simple lemon squeezer will do.
This simple recipe helps detoxify the liver; it works very well first thing in the morning.

Serves: 1
Ingredients:
- 2 lemons
- 1 tablespoon olive oil
- Pinch of Himalaya salt

Instructions:
1. Juice the lemons.
2. In a small glass, combine the lemon juice with the oil and Himalaya salt.
3. Stir well, say 3-2-1 and drink.
4. To your health!

(yea...sometimes it's about the taste, and sometimes it's about the benefit)

Avocado Oil – The Child of an Unusual Fruit

The avocado is a pretty amazing fruit! Why? Well, unlike most fruits, it's very rich in healthy fats and can be used to produce oil. It's not as well-known as olive oil or coconut oil, however, it's equally healthy and can be a fantastic addition to your alkaline keto smoothies, salads, and snacks.

Benefits of avocado oil:
-As much as 70% of avocado oil consists of oleic acid, which is great for heart health.

- It's high in lutein, a natural antioxidant that is great for maintaining healthy eyesight. Lutein may also lower the risk of age-related eye diseases.

-Helps essential nutrients absorb better
So important for all of us! I mean, what is the benefit of eating a super delicious salad if your body can't absorb the nutrients properly? Luckily, avocado oil can help. Many nutrients need fat to be absorbed better and faster by your body. This is why, it is recommended to drizzle some avocado oil to your salads or add it to your smoothies and juices.

-May improve joint health and decrease pain

Various studies have shown that extracts from avocado may reduce the stiffness and pain associated with osteoarthritis.

-Improved gum health
Extracts from avocado can prevent gum disease. This is because certain substances present in avocado and avocado oil may block an inflammation-provoking protein called IL1B, therefore protecting your gums.

-Helps neutralize free radicals
Antioxidants present in avocados and avocado oil, fight cellular damage caused by free radicals, which are waste products of metabolism. High levels of free radicals can lead to oxidative stress, therefore leading to diseases like type 2 diabetes and heart disease.

-Natural skin and hair moisturizer – avocado oil is a fabulous holistic beauty treatment, especially recommended for dry skin. It's also helpful to reduce wrinkles and give your skin a glowing, healthy look.

So how to add avocado oil to your diet?
-Add a tablespoon or two to a nutritious smoothie
-Drizzle over a big salad.
-Use it as a marinade for grilling meat.
-Use it to make hummus
-Drizzle it over cold soups, vegetable creams, and gazpacho (so yummy and healthy!)

Now, let's have a look at some delicious avocado oil recipes, including salads, smoothies, and juices. Then, we will also have a look at a few beauty and relaxation recipes, including avocado oil.

Spicy Ginger Salmon Salad

Ginger is well-known for its anti-inflammatory and healing properties. Cucumbers are highly refreshing and very alkaline-forming. Salmon, avocado, nuts, and healthy oils will help you stay full for hours!

Serves: 2
Ingredients
For the Salad:
- 2 cucumbers, peeled and thinly sliced
- 1 tablespoon of grated ginger
- 1 cup arugula leaves
- 1 big avocado, peeled, pitted and sliced
- A handful of crushed almonds
- 2 slices of smoked salmon, cut into smaller pieces

For the Dressing:
- 1 tablespoon avocado oil
- 1 tablespoon fresh lime juice
- Black pepper to taste
- Himalayan salt to taste

To garnish:
- A few orange wedges
- A handful of cilantro leaves

Instructions:
1. Combine all the salad ingredients in a big salad bowl and toss well.
2. Mix all the salad dressing ingredients. You can use a small hand blender, or quickly combine and stir all the ingredients in a small bowl.
3. Pour the dressing over the salad and toss well.
4. Sprinkle over a handful of cilantro leaves and garnish with orange wedges.
5. Serve and enjoy!

Quick Green Egg Salad

Hard-boiled eggs are quick time savers! They taste great in alkaline-keto salads and will help you stay full longer. Be sure to go for organic, free-range eggs.

Serves: 2
Ingredients:
For the Salad:
- 2 hard-boiled eggs
- ¼ cup of raw walnuts, chopped
- 1 small and ripe avocado (peeled and diced)
- 1 cup mixed leafy greens of your choice

For the Dressing:
- ½ teaspoon of freshly cracked black pepper
- 1 teaspoon of herbs de Provence
- ¼ teaspoon of Himalayan or sea salt
- 2 tablespoons of olive oil
- 2 tablespoons apple cider vinegar
- 2 tablespoons avocado oil

Instructions:
1. Boil the eggs.
2. In the meantime, combine all the salad ingredients in a big salad bowl.
3. Cooldown the boiled eggs by putting them in cold water.
4. Now, blend all the dressing ingredients using a small blender.
5. Peel the eggs and add them to the salad. Toss well.
6. Pour the salad dressing over the salad.
7. Toss well, serve and enjoy!

Pomegranate Avocado Anti-Sugar Cravings Juice

This recipe will help you get rid of sugar cravings while feeding your body with a myriad of nutrients it needs to thrive. Pomegranate juice is full of alkaline minerals as well as Vitamin C.
It's a natural antioxidant and anti-inflammatory. It blends well with ginger, turmeric, and mint. You can't juice avocado...but you can use avocado oil.

Servings: 2
Ingredients:
- 1 cup pomegranate
- 1-inch ginger root, peeled
- 1-inch turmeric root, peeled
- A handful of fresh mint leaves
- 2 tablespoons of avocado oil
- Stevia to sweeten (optional)

Procedure:
1. Juice the pomegranate, ginger, turmeric, and mint.
2. Combine with avocado oil.
3. Serve and enjoy!

Cucumber Kale Weight Loss Juice

While it's hard to eat a mountain of greens and cucumbers, it's easy to drink their juice and get all the vital nutrients from them. Avocado oil offers good fat to help you absorb the minerals and vitamins from the juice.

Servings: 2
Ingredients:
- 1 cup of kale, chopped
- 4 big cucumbers, peeled and chopped
- 2 limes, peeled
- 2 tablespoons of avocado oil
- Himalayan salt and black pepper to taste (optional)

Instructions:
1. Place through a juicer.
2. Pour into a glass and mix in some Himalayan salt and black pepper to taste. Stir in the avocado oil.
3. Enjoy!

Lime Refresher Ice Smoothie

This smoothie combines the best of alkaline keto fruits and herbs to help you enjoy energy and vitality. It's super refreshing as well!

Servings: 2

Ingredients

- 2 grapefruits, peeled and sliced
- 2 limes, peeled and sliced
- 1 tablespoon fresh oregano
- 1 cup almond milk
- 1 tablespoon avocado oil

Instructions:

1. Place all the ingredients in a blender.
2. Process well until smooth.
3. Serve and enjoy!

Simple Lemon Smoothie

This smoothie helps maintain a healthy digestive system. It's also great for detox.

Servings: 2
Ingredients:
- A handful of fresh mint leaves
- 1 lemon, peeled and sliced
- 1 cup water, filtered, preferably alkaline
- Pinch of Himalayan salt
- 2 tablespoons avocado oil

Instructions:
1. Place all the ingredients in a blender.
2. Process well until smooth.
3. Serve and enjoy!

Natural Relaxation Anti-Wrinkle Blend

Ingredients:

-1 tablespoon avocado oil

-2 drops lavender essential oil

-1 drop chamomile essential oil

Blend well and use it as a night moisturizer. Apply on washed and dried skin, enjoy the aroma, and relax!

Anti-Cellulite Blend

Ingredients:

-4 tablespoons avocado oil

-2 drops fennel essential oil

-2 drops lavender essential oil

Instructions:

Combine all the ingredients. Apply to your body via massage.

Enjoy! This blend is also great for relaxation!

Now, it's time to meet other oils!

Flaxseed Oil – From Health to Skin Care

Flax seeds offer many amazing health benefits such as a super-rich protein and fiber content, reducing sugar cravings, and natural weight loss.

No wonder that their child – flaxseed oil also offers a myriad of health and wellness benefits.

Flaxseed oil (also called flax oil or linseed oil), is made from ground and pressed flax seeds, and it can be used for many health and beauty treatments.

Benefits of Flaxseed Oil:

-Reduced inflammation, improved heart health, and brain protection due to the high content of Omega-3 fatty acids.

Flaxseed oil is an excellent natural Omega-3 supplement that is suitable for vegans and vegetarians. So, if, for some reason, you can't get fresh fish oil or fatty fish in your diet (or are not getting enough), try taking 1-2 tablespoons of flaxseed oil every day.

-Improved heart health

Several studies have shown that flaxseed oil could be very beneficial for heart health. It could even lead to lowering blood pressure. Another benefit of the flaxseed oil is that it could lead to improved elasticity of the arteries.

-Flaxseed oil may ease constipation and diarrhea- flaxseed oil can be very useful in increasing the frequency of bowel movements.

-Great for skin health - Flaxseed oil is very hydrating and soothing for the skin. It may also help reduce stretch marks and cellulite. Additionally, it can be used for scalp massage and as a natural hair conditioner. Simply massage your hair with flaxseed oil, keep it in for at least an hour and then wash your hair in a natural, gentle shampoo.

-Reduced inflammation – since flaxseed oil is very rich in omega-3 content, it may help reduce inflammation in some people, especially when combined with a healthy, clean, anti-inflammatory diets.

How to Use Flaxseed Oil to Unlock Its Health Benefits

The best way to use flaxseed oil is by adding it to salad dressings, dips, sauces, raw soups, and smoothies.

Unfortunately, flaxseed oil can't be used for cooking as it can form harmful compounds when exposed to high heat.

Additionally, you can use flaxseed oil for natural beauty treatments – it can be applied to the skin or as a hair mask.

Now, let's have a look at my favorite flaxseed oil recipes!

Pomegranate Alkaline Green Smoothie

Almonds make this smoothie taste amazing, and they also add in good fats and protein. Pomegranates are low in sugar and super high in alkaline minerals such as magnesium. They add an exciting twist to this green smoothie! Maca and Ashwagandha help you balance your hormones and feel less stressed.

Servings: 2-3
Ingredients
Liquid:
- 1 cup almond milk, unsweetened
- Half cup water, filtered, preferably alkaline
- 1 tablespoon flaxseed oil

Dry:
- Half cup pomegranates
- A handful of almonds
- Half cup spinach

Other:
- Stevia to sweeten, if desired
- Half teaspoon cinnamon powder
- Half teaspoon nutmeg powder

Instructions:
1. Place all the ingredients in a blender.
2. Process well until smooth.
3. Serve and enjoy!

Easy Hydration Mineral Green Smoothie

This is a super hydrating smoothie. It's jam-packed with energy restoring alkaline minerals and healthy fats. It's also rich in protein and will help you stay full for hours!

Servings: 2
Ingredients
Liquid:
- 1 cup water, filtered, preferably alkaline
- Half cup of coconut milk
- 1 tablespoon flaxseed oil

Dry:
- 1 big cucumber, peeled and chopped
- 1 zucchini, peeled and chopped (steamed or lightly cooked is preferred)
- 1 cup romaine lettuce, washed

Other:
- Himalaya salt to taste
- 1 tablespoon hemp seed or green pea protein powder

Instructions:
1. Place all the ingredients in a blender.
2. Process well until smooth.
3. Serve and enjoy!

Good Ol' Oil Green Smoothie

The delicious blend of sweet potatoes and spices makes it a perfect comfort smoothie. It also uses good fats and healthy protein to help you stay full for hours!

Serves 1-2

Ingredients:

Liquid:

- 1 cup coconut milk
- Half cup water, filtered, preferably alkaline
- 2 tablespoons flaxseed oil

Dry:

- 1 big sweet potato, peeled and cooked
- Half an avocado pitted and peeled
- A handful of cilantro leaves, washed
- A handful of parsley leaves, washed

Other:

- Pinch of Himalayan salt
- Pinch of curry powder
- Optional (if you like it spicy) a pinch of chili powder
- 1 teaspoon spirulina powder

Instructions:

1. Place all the ingredients in a blender.
2. Process until smooth.

3. Taste to check if you like to taste or if you need to add a bit more of Himalayan salt or curry powder

Serve in a smoothie glass, or a bowl and enjoy!

Brazil Nuts Quick Detox Salad

This recipe is a fantastic detox recipe as it's full of fresh, alkalizing ingredients and full of healing vitamins and minerals.

Serves: 2

Ingredients:
- 2 big cucumbers, peeled and sliced
- A handful or radish, halved
- A small garlic clove, minced
- A handful of raw Brazil nuts, roughly chopped
- 2 big tomatoes, sliced and peeled
- Juice of half lime
- 1 tablespoon of flaxseed oil
- Himalaya salt to taste
- Pinch of black pepper to taste

Instructions:
1. Place the cucumbers, radish, and tomatoes in a salad bowl.
2. Add Brazil nuts and garlic.
3. Sprinkle over some olive oil, lime juice, Himalaya salt, and black pepper to taste.
4. Toss well and enjoy!

Easy Mediterranean Salad

This salad is more than just a "green salad". It's a simple yet sophisticated blend of healing Mediterranean spices, and unique taste you will surely get hooked on. The best part? It's very easy to make.

Serves: 2-3
Ingredients:
- Half cup of fresh basil leaves
- 1 cup of fresh cherry tomatoes, halved
- 1 cup of arugula leaves
- A handful of baby spinach leaves
- Half cup of black olives, pitted
- Half cup of green olives, pitted
- ¼ cup of raw pine nuts
- 1 tablespoon of flaxseed oil
- Himalaya salt to taste.
- feta cheese (optional)

Instructions:
1. In a salad bowl combine the fresh basil leaves, cherry tomatoes, arugula leaves, handful of spinach leaves, olives, and pine nuts.
2. Toss well. Add some feta cheese if needed.
3. Now, sprinkle over some olive oil and Himalaya salt to taste if needed.
4. Toss again, serve, and enjoy!

Easy Chilly Beetroot Soup

This soup is creamy, comforting, and very easy to make. Such a great way of sneaking in some flaxseed oil!

Servings: 2-3

Ingredients:

- 1 small avocado peeled and pitted
- 1 small beetroot, peeled and chopped
- 2 tablespoons of spring onion, chopped
- 1 small cucumber, peeled
- Half green apple, chopped
- 1 cup water, filtered, preferably alkaline
- Half cup almond or coconut milk
- 2 tablespoons flaxseed oil

Toppings:

- Fresh dill, chive or herbs like oregano
- Crushed nuts

Instructions:

1. Add all ingredients to blender.
2. Blend well until smooth.
3. Taste and adjust seasonings if needed. Blend together once again.
4. Serve room temperature or chilled. Add toppings of your choice.

Aromatherapy & Essential Oil Recipes for Beauty & Health

Water Retention Killers

If you feel like water retention is killing you, try this mix:

Blend:

2 tablespoons of flaxseed oil

5 drops of juniper essential oil +

2 drops of peppermint essential oil+

5 drops of geranium essential oil

Apply as a full body massage. You will experience immediate relief.

Mint is refreshing and cooling. Juniper and geranium have some really great detoxifying properties, and they also stimulate venous circulation.

Beautiful Skin

This is a very simple blend that can be applied to all kinds of skins.

Blend:

1 tablespoon of flaxseed oil +

1 drop of geranium essential oil +

1 drop of ylang ylang

To apply:

Gentle, facial massage.

Acne Killers

The following recipe is an excellent natural acne remedy.

This is a strong concentration blend and should be applied once or twice a day on acne affected areas.

Blend:

1 tablespoon flaxseed oil

1 drop of palmarosa essential oil +

1 drop of tea tree essential oil +

1 drop of lavender essential oil

Apply on the skin through a gentle massage.

Aroma Moisturizers

If you suffer from dry or chapped skin, this is the blend for you.

Blend:

2 tablespoons of flaxseed oil+

2 drops of lavandin+

1 drop of ylang-ylang+

2 drops of jasmine+

2 drops of German (or Roman) Chamomile

Apply:

Apply as a full-body massage, you can also use it on your face, but I suggest you test a small area first if you have extremely sensitive skin.

Sesame Oil – the Ancient Ayurveda Miracle

Sesame oil is a child of raw, pressed sesame seeds. It has multiple culinary, medicinal, and even cosmetic uses. It's also very popular among yogis, as well as in traditional Ayurvedic medicine. It's also commonly used in the macrobiotic diet.

Let's have at its amazing health benefits:

-High in antioxidants - Sesame oil is very rich in sesamol which is a very powerful antioxidant that helps reduce cell damage caused by free radicals. By reducing free radicals, you reduce inflammation and decrease the risk of disease.

Sesame oil can have similar benefits, also when applied topically. It's also commonly used for therapeutic massages, especially in traditional, Ayurvedic spas.

-Offers strong anti-inflammatory properties – sesame oil has been used in Oriental medicine, such as traditional Taiwanese medicine for years. Its most common uses include treating joint inflammation, scrapes, and even toothaches.

-Great for improved heart health – sesame oil consists of more than 80% unsaturated fatty acids, and it's especially rich in omega-6 fatty acids. These are polyunsaturated fats that are very important to your diet and can prevent heart disease.

-May be beneficial for controlling blood sugar - Sesame oil can help support healthy blood sugar regulation, and it can be a great addition to your smoothies.

-Wound and burn healing – sesame oil can also be used topically for wounds and burns. Since it's very rich in antioxidants and anti-inflammatory properties, it can speed up wound healing.

-Natural sun protection – sesame oil can protect against the harmful UV rays, to a certain degree. Other oils, such as coconut oil, can resist only 20% of UV rays, whereas sesame oil can go as far as up to 30% protection.

-Great for natural health treatments – compounds found in sesame oil can improve hair health, making it stronger and giving it more shine. This can be achieved by taking sesame oil as a supplement, as well as using it topically, as a hair mask, or for scalp massage.

How to add sesame oil to your diet

Sesame oil has a nice, natural, nutty flavor, and it's very often used in Asian and Middle Eastern cuisine.

Sesame Oil Secrets

There are different kinds of sesame oil:

-Unrefined is light in color, has a very nutty flavor, and can be used for cooking (low to medium heat).

-Refined sesame oil is more processed, therefore, has fewer health benefits. It's flavor is more neutral and, in Asian and Oriental cuisine, it's commonly used for deep- or stir-frying.

-Toasted sesame oil is famous for its brown color as well as delicate flavor, and it's widely used for salad dressings and marinades.

Sesame oil is usually used for:

-stir-fries

-marinades

-vinaigrettes

-sauces, dips or soups

Sesame Oil Recipes

Tahini Sesame Energy Soup

If you always crave sugar and processed foods, adding more good fats such as tahini and sesame oil can make a difference.

Servings: 2

Ingredients:

- 1 large handful of arugula leaves
- Juice of 1 lime
- 1 cup coconut or cashew milk
- Half cup of water
- 3 dates, peeled and pitted
- 1 cucumber, peeled and pitted
- 1 big bell pepper, cut into smaller pieces
- 3 tablespoons of raw tahini
- 2 tablespoons sesame oil
- 1 small avocado, peeled and pitted
- Himalayan salt to taste
- Optional: cilantro and parsley to garnish

Instructions:

1. Add all ingredients to a blender. Blend well until smooth.
2. Add more water to or coconut/cashew milk, if needed.
3. Serve and enjoy!

Power Sesame Smoothie

If you are looking for a smoothie to replace a meal, or to have a snack, try this nutritious smoothie!

Ingredients:

- 4 cubes of frozen spinach
- half small roasted pumpkin
- half avocado, peeled and pitted
- 1 cup of coconut water
- 1 tablespoon sesame oil
- 1 tablespoon sesame seeds
- 2 nori sheets

Instructions:

1. Place all of the ingredients in a blender.
2. Process well until smooth, serve and enjoy!

Spicy Mediterranean Smoothie

This smoothie is rich in good fats and protein and can be turned into a delicious, satisfying raw (or lightly cooked) soup.

Servings: 2
Ingredients:
- 2 green bell peppers, chopped, seeds removed
- Half avocado, peeled and pitted
- 1 small garlic clove, peeled
- Pinch of black pepper and chili
- 1 cup almond milk, unsweetened
- A handful of almonds, soaked in water for at least a few hours
- 1 tablespoon sesame oil
- Himalaya salt to taste

Instructions:
1. Place all the ingredients in a blender.
2. Process until smooth, serve, and enjoy!

Mood Boosting Smoothie

Having a bad day? Do you need to boost your mood? Try this smoothie. It offers a healthy mix of vitamin C, energy stimulating greens, and mood-boosting cocoa.

Servings: 1-2
Ingredients:
Liquid:
- 1 cup of coconut milk
- Half cup water, filtered
- 1 tablespoon sesame oil

Dry:
- 1-inch ginger, peeled
- 1-inch turmeric, peeled
- Half cup arugula leaves
- 1 orange, peeled

Other:
- Stevia to sweeten (optional)
- Half teaspoon cinnamon
- 1 tablespoon cocoa powder
- 1 tablespoon chia seeds
- A few drops of liquid chlorophyll

Instructions:
1. Blend and enjoy.
2. Add some stevia to sweeten if needed.
3. This drink is great first thing in the morning. But you can also sip on it during the day to enjoy more energy or whenever you are having a bad day!

Healing Ashwagandha Juice

Ashwagandha powder is a great choice to help you re-balance your energy levels while feeling more relaxed. Coconut milk makes this juice creamy and soft.

Servings: 2
Ingredients:
- 2 red bell peppers, chopped
- 1 lime, peeled and chopped
- 1 cup of coconut milk
- 2 tablespoons sesame oil
- Half teaspoon Ashwagandha powder

Instructions:
1. Juice the bell peppers and lime.
2. Pour into a small hand blender and combine with coconut milk, sesame oil, and Ashwagandha.
3. Blend until smooth and creamy.

Pour into a glass and enjoy!

Oriental Alkaline Keto Green Salad

This salad is perfect for a quick detox (or alkaline cleanse), or as a side dish!

Serves:2
Ingredients:
Salad:
- 1 cup of fresh spring greens
- 2 handfuls of fresh basil leaves, torn roughly
- 5oz. (150 grams) of fresh cherry tomatoes cut in halves
- 1 whole avocado, peeled, pitted and sliced

For the Dressing:
- 1 tablespoon of sesame oil
- A pinch of ground cumin
- 2 tablespoons of fresh lemon juice
- 1 teaspoon curry powder
- A pinch of Himalayan salt
- Half teaspoon of ground coriander

To Garnish:
- A few fresh mint, parsley, and cilantro leaves

Instructions:
1. Combine all the salad ingredients in a big salad bowl and toss well.
2. Mix all the salad dressing ingredients.
3. Pour the dressing over the salad and stir well.
4. Sprinkle over a few mint, parsley, and cilantro leaves. Enjoy!

Easy Spinach'n' Nuts Salad

This simple plant-based alkaline keto salad is excellent for detox. It can also be served as a simple side dish to help you incorporate more greens into your diet.

Serves:2
Ingredients
For the Salad:
- 2 cups of fresh strawberries, sliced
- 1 cup of fresh baby spinach
- 4 tablespoons of chopped walnuts
- 1 big avocado, peeled, pitted and sliced

Dressing:
- 1 tablespoon of coconut vinegar
- 4 tablespoons of sesame oil
- Some pepper and Himalayan salt to taste

Instructions:
1. Whisk the sesame oil, coconut vinegar, ground black pepper, and sea salt in a bowl until the dressing becomes smooth, and you get a well-combined dressing.
2. Slice the strawberries, chop the walnuts, and slice the avocado.
3. Combine the spinach with walnuts, strawberries, and avocado and drizzle the prepared dressing over the salad.
4. Toss the salad lightly to mix well and serve immediately. Enjoy!

Hair & Scalp Massage Recipe

Blend:

-4 tablespoons of sesame oil

-4 drops of lavender essential oil

-2 drops of lemon essential oil

Massage into the scalp. Keep massaging for at least a few minutes. Leave in for at least 1 hour and wash out with a gentle shampoo. Enjoy, it's very relaxing!

Anti-Age Sesame Oil Face Mask

Blend:
-2 tablespoons sesame oil
-3 tablespoons honey
-2 drops of lavender essential oil

Apply and leave in for 20 minutes. Wash with warm water and moisturize if needed.

Ayurvedic Sesame Body Scrub

Blend:

-4 tablespoons sesame oil

-4 tablespoons Epsom salt

-2 drops of sandalwood essential oil

Blend all the ingredients, place in a bowl, and use it as a natural body peeling or scrub whenever needed.

Relaxation and Meditation Oil Blend

This blend is my favorite relaxation blend! I love to use it after a nice, relaxing Epsom salt bath, or before my evening meditation.

Blend:

-2 tablespoons sesame oil

-2 drops of ylang-ylang or rose essential oil

Blend the oils and use as massage oil (avoid the eye area). Enjoy!

More Alkaline Keto Books

Join Our VIP Readers' Newsletter to Boost Your Wellbeing

Would you like to be notified about our new health and wellness books? How about receiving them at deeply discounted prices?

What about awesome giveaways, latest health tips, and motivation?

If that is something you are interested in, please visit the link below to join our newsletter:

www.yourwellnessbooks.com/email-newsletter

As a bonus, you will receive a free complimentary eBook *Alkaline Paleo Superfoods*

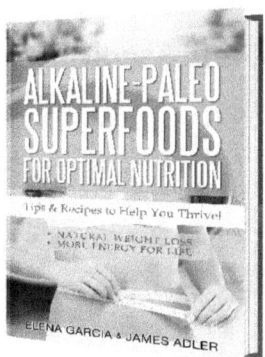

Sign up link:

www.yourwellnessbooks.com/email-newsletter

(any technical problems with your sign up, please email: info@yourwellnessbooks.com)

More Books & Resources in the Healthy Lifestyle Series
Available at:

www.yourwellnessbooks.com

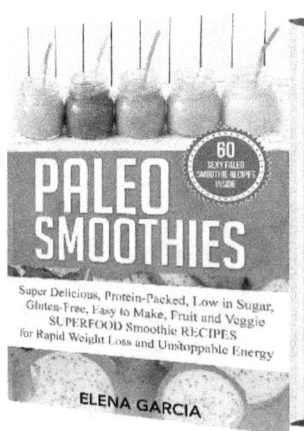
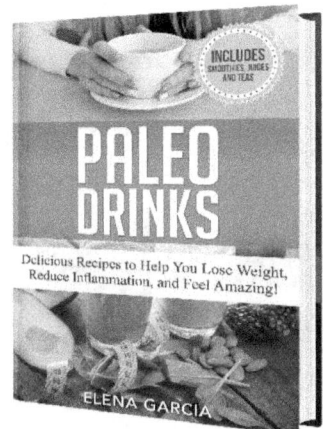
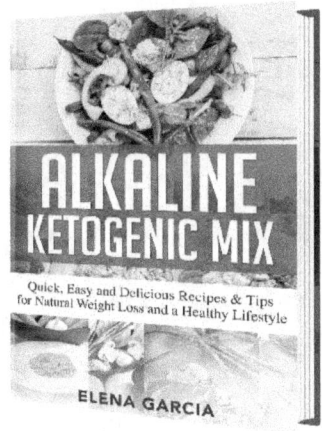
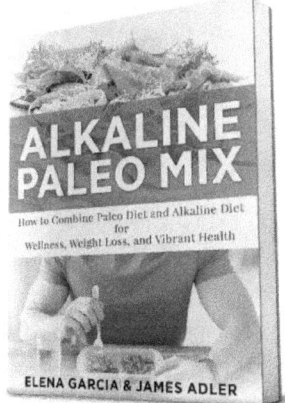

More Alkaline Keto Books

Until next time, wishing you all the best on your journey!

Elena & Your Wellness Books Team

www.YourWellnessBooks.com

We Need Your Help

One more thing, before you go, could you please do us a quick favor?

It would be great if you could leave us a short review on Amazon.

Don't worry, it doesn't have to be long. One sentence is enough.

Let others know your favorite recipes and who you think this book can help.

Your review can inspire more and more people to turn to the alkaline ketogenic lifestyle so that they can finally achieve their wellness and weight loss goals the way they deserve.

Your honest review is critical.

Thank You for your support!

More Alkaline Keto Books

www.ingramcontent.com/pod-product-compliance
Lightning Source LLC
Chambersburg PA
CBHW071407080526
44587CB00017B/3197